Home Based Workout for Women

30+ Exercises to Make Your Body Lean with Homebased Workout. Reduce Fat by Doing Aerobics, Zumba and Planks

By

Hazel M.

Disclaimer Notice

This book is written and published independently. Please keep in mind that the material in this publication is solely for educational and entertaining purposes. All efforts have provided authentic, up-to-date, trustworthy, and comprehensive information. There are no express or implied assurances. The purpose of this book's material is to assist readers in having a better understanding of the subject matter. The activities, information, and exercises are provided solely for self-help information. This book is not intended to replace expert psychologists, legal, financial, or other guidance. If you require counseling, please get in touch with a qualified professional.

By reading this text, the reader accepts that the author will not be held liable for any damages, indirectly or directly, experienced due to the use of the information included herein, particularly, but not limited to, omissions, errors, or inaccuracies. As a reader, you are accountable for your decisions, actions, and consequences.

About the Author

Hazel M. is a dedicated advocate for women's health and a certified fitness instructor renowned for her Zumba, planks, and aerobics expertise. With over a decade of experience in the fitness industry, Hazel's passion lies in helping women to embrace their strength and transform their lives through exercise. Her book, "Home-Based Workout for Women," is a comprehensive guide that inspires and equips women of all backgrounds to have a fitness regime from the comfort of their homes.

Through her uplifting and practical approach, Hazel aims to help women build stronger bodies and a resilient mindset, fostering a sense of confidence and accomplishment in every reader. Whether a seasoned fitness enthusiast or a newcomer, her book is your ultimate companion to reach your potential and achieve a healthier, fitter, and more empowered you.

Contents

Introduction

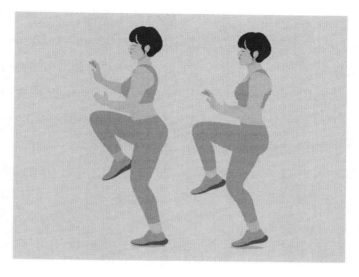

At one point in my life, I felt more hopelessness than I had ever handled. I was at my lowest point. It felt a total lack of control. I had a strong sense of resolve at that very moment. When my spiritual guru failed to help me materialize my goal, I decided to become my own guru.

I spent the following years researching and analyzing each workout and diet available. I devoured every significant book, read countless academic papers, and attended workshops. I collaborated with psychiatrists, dietitians, physical therapists, and doctors. I had a strong feeling of purpose.

According to research, small, regular lifestyle adjustments are the most effective method to transform habits in a real, long-lasting way. After making several significant lifestyle changes, I was feeling fairly good. However, a perfect storm struck one day, and I once more found myself at the emotional bottom. I had family issues, and I felt entirely alone. Have you ever encountered such a deluge of disappointments? I was not the embodiment of empowerment and well-being that I wanted to be. This made me take a close look at myself once more.

Meet the New 'Me'

I came home from a long day of work. I was hungry and exhausted, and it was raining heavily. Yet I had vowed to begin a new exercise regimen and permanently lose weight.

There was no way around it—I needed to drag myself to my new gym immediately!

It was already late by the time I had checked the kids into childcare and put their belongings into the room. I entered the crowded gym only to discover that every machine was occupied. I considered using the free weights but ultimately scratched that idea.

I waited for long. I eventually completed my final set of the evening, picked up the kids, and then trekked back to my car through the pouring rain again. My husband complained about me being late for dinner.

Everyone who wants to get in shape eventually has to deal with the inconveniences of these routines and gyms. That turns off many women to the point where their fitness plans are derailed. But things don't need to stay like that.

What if you could go into your basement and work out quickly while your children do their work? You wouldn't have to put on makeup or style your hair; you could wear whatever you wanted and listen to music you wanted. No need to drive in bad weather. No waiting in line for machines. No need to be concerned about contaminated equipment. No heavy machines to get a lean body.

Own your home workout space. One word best describes the advantages of having your home gym: independence. You are free to act, however, whenever you like. Naturally, you are exempt from paying the expensive membership dues, which can total thousands of dollars annually. This book is an excellent tool for taking you through that process if you've decided that a home-based workout is the best option.

How to Use this Book?

I have assisted several ladies in designing their home-based workout plans and demonstrating the best ways to use different exercises to reach their fitness objectives. I will do it for you in the pages that come after. This book will show you how you can achieve the target of reducing your extra fats whether you are beginning from scratch, improving an existing home-based workout regime, or simply trying to change what you already have.

Chapter one sets your foundation and a mindset to begin your journey. In chapter two, you will learn tips on selecting an exercise location, making the most of your available area, and getting long-lasting results. Many women spend a lot of money on unnecessary fancy items. Ultimately, they receive a much lower price for these items when they trade them in or sell them. You can prevent this issue by using the advice in these chapters.

You can always have a few workout options, regardless of whether you've only recently decided to enter the weight room or have been working out for some time.

This book fills that need. You can find a routine for every requirement and any day of the week, whether you want an entire lean body at once or concentrate on just one body part. This book can be applied in a variety of ways.

Your workout regimen should be varied, or it could concentrate on a certain body component that needs attention. Sometimes, trying something new is how to get yourself moving and combat monotony. If you are tired of planks, go to the chapter on Zumba dance and pick on aerobics exercises. However, if your shoulders aren't creating the cap that makes your hips and waist appear smaller, give them a push.

Choose a leg workout from Chapter six, and perform each one on alternate days of the week. You've just designed your very own full-body workout regimen.

You may want to change your exercise regimen. Try some new exercises in that case. This book contains 35+ illustrated exercises so that you can replace one or two of your existing workouts with a few.

Overall, this book has workouts that would take years to complete. It might be the best fitness resource you've ever had. In short, this book offers a thorough guide for designing the ideal home workout regime. If you heed the suggestions, you will have the know-how and resources to create a unique workout plan for years of lasting enjoyment and a lean physique.

Chapter 1: You Go, Girl!

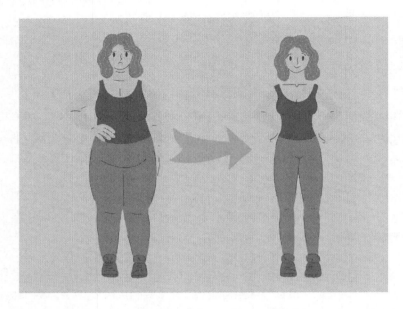

I had tried all methods and plans when struggling with my weight. I had never been engaged in an exercise intended to build my physical strength. I would certainly lift weights, enter the gym, and perform a few exercises, but I had never been trained for strength as one should. Then, I chose a home-based workout with Zumba, planks, and aerobics because it was the only one left.

A part of me understood that developing an extraordinarily robust physical life would not be easy. I had the impression that I knew I would develop emotional toughness through strength training. My home-based workout routine would help me get my ideal physique and strengthen me.

I had to wait approximately a year to see real changes in my body. That year was undoubtedly the most difficult year, in an oddly beautiful sense. I had intended to reconstruct my physique, but instead, I ended myself physically, emotionally, mentally, and spiritually reinventing my entire existence.

My life metaphor was my home-based gym. I had to push through the difficult periods since I was committed to improving my body, and those challenging moments forced me to consider my motives and the justifications I had been using for myself. Lean body and weight loss helped me regain my strength after I had been emotionally battered.

I overcame my dependence on sugar and caffeine and naturally treated my knees. I became aware of how awful I was for my entire adult life. My life changed. The only words I could say to myself then were, 'You Go, Girl!'

1.1 A Lean Body: Meet Your Empowered Self

I've observed an intriguing tendency in females I have interacted in my life. The most frequent reaction I get when I probe further into their motivations for visiting me is that they want to appear better and lose weight. They look ashamed when they tell me this, and some of them make comments about how they feel vain to express it.

As we discuss this further, they admit that they don't care about their appearance and that society sees vanity as a selfish and destructive motivation. They appear to be ashamed of their desire to look better.

Acceptance is crucial: It's normal to desire to feel confident in your appearance. You should be proud of yourself because trying to look good and lean is a show of self-respect. Be proud of your vanity and own it. You are to be commended for having the guts to declare, " I'm going to have a healthy body."

Yet, trying to please other people will never be enough. It should not be the inspiration for a significant and long-lasting transformation. You want a long-lasting change. That's why you need this book.

What Are Your Shackles?

Why have you yet to fulfil your fitness vision? There are two reasons why most women haven't gotten their ideal bodies.

1. They lack the knowledge necessary to carry it out because they have yet to discover a method that works.

2. They are bothered by the notion that their only motivation is avarice.

But why they don't have the bodies they desire; they typically give one of these three excuses:

◊   They are Lazy

Would you describe yourself as lazy if you examined every aspect of your life? Are there any aspects of your life that you absolutely detest? If so, you aren't idle. You may struggle with fitness motivation, but you are not inattentive.

◊   They don't want it badly enough.

Do you have a strong energy when you picture your lean body? Then you really do want it. You don't know how to achieve that without excruciatingly difficult exercises, long cardio sessions, or a diet that makes you a hangry grump monster. You may long for your ideal body but don't know how to get it. Yet.

◊ Their bodies are "quirky" and don't appear to respond well to exercise.

Have you ever experienced a time when you were truly satisfied with your physical appearance or level of fitness? Have you ever had an exercise regimen and had positive results? If so, this is evidence that your body is set up to respond positively to your food and exercise efforts. You are not as eccentric as you believe! You've already done it, so you do it once more.

You haven't found a method that works for your body or perhaps you need the proper motives, causing you to discontinue a program before it has a chance to make a difference. You will discover the answers to your problems in the upcoming chapters. You will also learn to find the answers that work for you because everyone is unique.

Your body's status is something you can control. You can design the physique of your desires. You can lose weight, get leaner, and ultimately meet 'Your Empowered Self.'

1.2 Your Mindset Matters

I know the factors that contribute to women's success in transforming their bodies. Some women have succeeded in getting their dream bodies because they are in touch with their true motivations. However, for many women, including myself, some standards symbolize our respect for our bodies. It is the idea that it is our responsibility to make the most of them. We engage in it because it embodies who we are, advances our development, and allows us to explore fully.

Because I finally realized that I could achieve what I wanted for myself, I was able to transform my life and reach a higher level of fitness.

You need greater energy, intelligence, or intuition. I have to acknowledge my own deserving of such brilliance. Those who are exceptional are distinguished by their conviction that they deserve greatness, their capacity to realize it, and their prodigious effort. They develop their superpowers, in other words. You can do the same and have the right mindset.

The idea that changing one's body is simple is one of the biggest fallacies in health and fitness. Making lasting changes and being healthy is difficult. Everyone would be fit if it were simple, right?

Discipline is necessary for getting fit. I've discovered that these human characteristics are the most challenging. Sometimes, you must push through fatigue, exert effort when you don't want to, and stand when you'd rather sit down to get fitter.

Because of this, most women are not motivated by vanity, so you must have connections to stronger forces at work in the world. You will think when the day arrives (and it will) when you are expected to get up and hit your home-based gym to work out, but you are not feeling it. Your vanity disappears when you are worn out, under pressure, or pushed for time.

You need potent motives to conquer these challenges and build the physique of your desires. Your higher self must serve as your motivation. Our accomplishments give us superpowers. They result from overcoming challenges and difficulties. It embodies the spirit of the human being. Resilience builds in the face of adversity.

Go deep, work hard, and stay the course—even when you don't feel like it—to achieve rock-solid empowerment and unwavering self-respect. And doing that will be a lot simpler if you are driven by something more than your appearance.

Only by creating your greatest "you" can you build your best body.

Now I can say this with absolute certainty: Getting the body you desire is feasible. I swear to you. Trust in my confidence, and don't question your abilities. You will experience amazing results if you believe in my belief in your abilities. Trust me. You can achieve anything you set out to do for yourself.

You must act!

Finding your motivations can be helpful, but ultimately, getting a lean body is just a matter of doing it. Simply put, you need to take massive action. A moving object usually continues to move. You must take action to overcome inertia and bring about this outcome for yourself.

I want you to experience the thrill of learning that you have developed an empowered self. This aspect of you is in charge of developing a physical manifestation of your inner excellence.

You will embark on a home-based workout journey with this book's help to develop a more profound sense of who you are. You will undergo so many amazing changes due to changing your body.

We will do it in a dancing and fun way. If you fully commit to following it, you will complete this book with a strong sense of accomplishment, resilience, and physical and personal strength. Building a lean and healthy body is simple when you take this approach. But hear me out: action is the key!

1.3 Why Does Reducing Fat Matter to Your Health?

The presence of fat is essential for the production of certain bodily processes, including hormone production and insulation. But having too much body fat can harm a woman's health and increase her risk for various illnesses, such as diabetes, heart disease, and some cancers.

Women can lower their risk of developing heart disease and improve their cardiovascular health by reducing fat through a healthy diet and consistent exercise.

Fat loss can aid in preventing type 2 diabetes, a chronic disease that millions of women worldwide are affected by. Insulin resistance is when the body's cells lose their sensitivity to the hormone insulin, which controls blood sugar levels. Excess fat can cause this condition. Type 2 diabetes and high sugar levels may result from this. Women can avoid both of them by losing fat.

Furthermore, your general quality of life can be enhanced by losing weight. Excessive fat can cause joint pain, mobility issues, and other health problems, making it difficult for women to perform daily tasks. Your mobility, joint pain, and general quality of life can all be improved by losing fat.

The mental health of a woman can benefit from losing fat as well. Low self-esteem, a negative body image, and depression can be brought on by excess fat. By losing fat, women's mental health, body image, and self-confidence can all be enhanced.

Reduced fat can assist women in maintaining a healthy weight in addition to the advantages to physical and mental health. Weight gain brought on by excess fat can raise a woman's risk of developing several health issues. Women can maintain a healthy weight and enhance their general health and well-being by reducing fat.

You should concentrate on leading healthy lifestyles, such as eating a diet high in vegetables, fruits, lean proteins, and whole grains and frequently exercising to lose weight. It is critical to understand that losing weight does not mean trying to achieve an unattainable or unhealthy body type. Instead, healthy weight should be maintained, and extra fat should be reduced to enhance overall health and well-being.

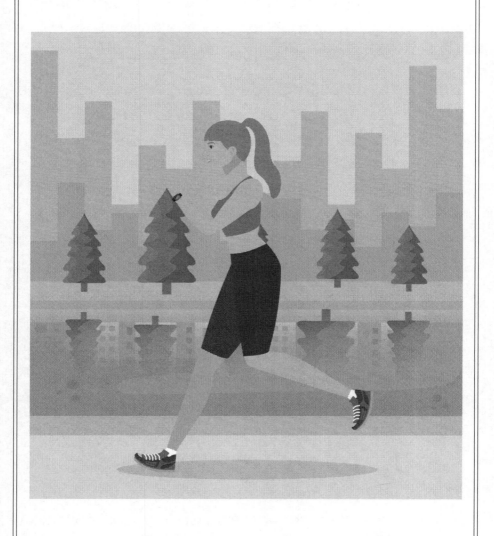

Chapter 2: Set the Stage

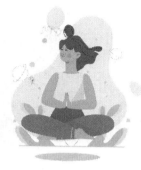

You've shown that you are committed to designing a home workout plan and beginning your exercise regimen by picking up this book. If so, that's fantastic. You require enthusiasm and persistence for success. However, think twice before you spend your hard-earned money on any item required.

Home gyms are too frequently built on the spur of the moment. Women might build high-tech exercise machines after seeing an advertisement, and they then hope to build the body of their dreams using a hurriedly put-together regimen. Regrettably, it is unlikely that this scenario will lead to the intended outcomes. You need a strategy if you want to do things correctly. In this book, we will explore aerobics, Zumba, and planks for your weight loss journey. For that, you do not need heavy machinery. I will demonstrate how to do it for you.

2.1 Finding a Space for Your Stage

Having said that, you can benefit greatly from giving your workout space extra room. To determine how to utilize your space most effectively for your purposes, ask yourself the following questions:

How much room can you set aside for your exercises?

Well, it depends on the type of exercise you are going to do and the equipment needed. Choose a place where there are no distractions. Make every attempt to keep your workout space away from where the kids are playing hide-and-seek or where your spouse is relaxing. You won't get a good workout in either of these locations, and they will also leave you anxious and stressed out, which is not a nice way to end an exercise session.

Does the space have enough insulation and ventilation?

Working out in an overly hot or humid environment depletes your strength and vitality, which lowers the effectiveness of your workout. In severe circumstances, you can experience heat stroke or possibly lose consciousness. Avoid taking chances. Ensure sure the space is properly aired. Install a sizable fan. During the chilly winter, the space should be adequately heated. Exercise performance and sufficient circulation are both hampered by extreme cold.

You should insulate the ceilings and walls if you intend to convert your garage into your working space. As you consider the layout of your home or apartment in light of your responses to these queries, consider which space could be most appropriate for your home gym. Be innovative.

2.2 Equipment Selection

Like I told you that you do not need fancy equipment for your workout. You need space to stretch, jump, dance, and enjoy! You will need a water bottle to stay hydrated, supportive sneakers, and cozy training attire for Zumba. Also, some women enjoy wearing sweatbands or wristbands to prevent sweat from dripping into their eyes. You don't need any special equipment to perform planks, but you might want a yoga mat or other soft surface to protect your knees and elbows.

You will need durable sneakers, a water bottle, and comfortable workout attire for aerobic workouts. Some women want to intensify their workouts by using resistance bands or hand weights. Overall, only a few basic pieces of equipment are required for these workouts, and the majority of women may begin with them.

Stability Ball

The stability ball is one of the most essential tools in a personal trainer's toolbox. Nobody can question the usefulness of stability balls as a training tool, thus you should utilize them in your home workout regime.

Stability balls are just huge, inflated balls that may be used for a variety of exercises. They are elegant in their simplicity. A ball can be used for any activity on a bench. Even better, its air-filled design adapts to the specific contours of your body.

Ball training adds some enjoyment to your regimen. Your body's inherent motor reflexes are stimulated to maintain good posture and alignment as a result of your core being forced into a stabilizing position. Research has shown that exercising on uneven surfaces significantly increases the amount of core activity. The evidence is quite strong.

The best approach is to train on a variety of surfaces, both stable and unsteady. An important part of your regimen should include ball exercises, for instance, if you wish to increase core activation.

The routines in the coming chapters will show you how this idea is applied.

Stability balls are available in various sizes. Another key consideration is your body type, particularly in light of your leg length. Your thighs have to be level with the floor. The ball is too big if your thighs slope downward; the opposite is true if your thighs slope upward.

Dumb shells

These are the most adaptable piece of home gym equipment. Dumbbells are known as free weights because they aren't connected to any machines. These enable you to carry out countless training modifications for each and every conceivable muscle area. Even better, they can be adjusted to fit any body type. You will never have a problem getting a fantastic workout with free weights.

Free weights allow you to develop your muscles in three dimensions, which is their best advantage. Most of the equipment needs to provide this complete freedom of motion.

Why is movement freedom during exercise so crucial? It resembles real-life activity. You move your body in order to pick up a parcel, move furniture, or accomplish any physical task. Free weight training enhances your capacity to carry out these duties in a way that machines cannot imitate. The ability to move freely has significant effects on body shaping, too.

Your body will look more polished and have superior muscle strength as a result. In short, free weights are a requirement if you want to maximize shape and symmetry; they are not an alternative.

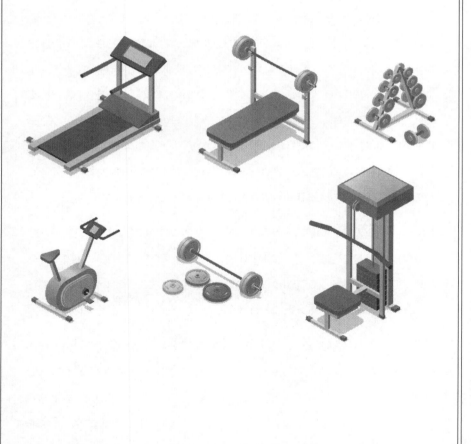

2.3 Fat Burning with Workout at Home

Do you need to shed off a few more pounds? Maybe more than one? If so, you should try your best at-home fat loss routine. It's a vigorous aerobic, plank, and Zumba routine meant to burn off extra pounds without affecting the lean muscle. The exercise variables are set up to bring change in intensity, duration, and mode in order to prevent repetition. You won't become bored since you will always be challenged.

You probably expect me to give you the usual advice, urging you to get to do a workout for an hour straight in your fat-burning zone. Zero chance! The fat-burning zone doesn't actually exist. The misconception is based on a misunderstanding of studies that indicate that during low-intensity exercise, the body prefers to use fat as fuel. Weight loss is the result of the number of calories burned overall, not just the proportion of calories from fat.

Aerobic exercise has no intrinsic flaws. It unquestionably aids in weight loss and overall cardiorespiratory health improvement. A great method to get the benefits of aerobic exercise without putting in a lot of physical effort is to exercise slowly. The most crucial part of the exercise is adherence. Choose steady-state cardio if you don't like doing high-intensity exercise or if a medical condition prevents you from doing intense training. Nonetheless, vigorous aerobic exercise is unquestionably your greatest bet for maximizing fat burning.

With the exercise given in this book, you will transform your body into a perpetual fat-burning machine that can keep you trimmed.

You will increase your muscle and fat cells' sensitivity to chemicals that help you lose weight, such as adrenaline, which aids in transferring fatty acids that can be used as fuel. Another illustration is insulin, which enables glucose to be transported to fat cells as lipids rather than being stored as glycogen in muscle tissues.

Your mitochondria, the cell's internal power factories that burn fat, will grow in size and quantity. This implies that you have long-term weight management. The number of enzymes available to catalyze metabolism will increase.

Even while all of these items work together to burn fat effectively, there is a catch. To maintain effects over time, these exercises must be paired with each other.

Why is maintaining muscle mass so crucial for weight loss?

If you are relaxing on the couch and watching your favorite TV show, you will burn more calories. Hence, your metabolism is slowed down as you lose muscle. Over time, this makes it harder to lose extra weight, inexorably resulting in a weight-loss journey. You start to feel frustrated, the weight starts to sneak back, and you become heavier than when you started.

Our sole purpose is to maintain muscular mass. Aerobic exercises not only slow down muscle loss, but they can also lead to an increase in muscle size. The metabolism remains high, weight loss is accelerated, and you get a lean body.

Rated Perceived Exertion (RPE) is an additional useful tool to evaluate the perceived exertion. This 10-point scale helps you subjectively estimate your exercise intensity. Learn what it's like to exercise at your fitness level. That's where I want you to spend the majority of your time exercising when you do Zumba.

This is the RPE graph:

The scale of Perceived exertion

1. Extremely simple: This is nearly like relaxation.

2. Easy: You experience this when you go about your regular tasks, such as getting dressed and so forth.

3. Quite simple. You experience this while moving from one location to another. The level of your respiration starts to rise, although only slightly.

4. Medium. Your breathing is getting deeper while you work at around half your maximum capacity.

5. Quite challenging: This resembles going for a brisk walk or performing a light exercise. Your breathing has become deeper. Making an effort to converse is necessary. You will experience this if you increase the speed of your brisk stroll. You are breathing more deeply, making it more difficult to maintain a conversation. You can continue to put in this amount of work for some time.

6. A little challenging. You are now engaging in an intense workout. Your heart is beating rapidly, and you are breathing deeply. It takes a lot of work to talk.

7. zHard: At this difficulty level, it feels like an extremely arduous task. You are inhaling deeply. Maintaining a conversation is challenging.

8. Extremely challenging. You are undoubtedly exerting a great deal of effort, which may cause you to feel really exhausted. You have trouble breathing, making it difficult to communicate. Most elite athletes train at this level.

9. Most challenging: This level necessitates an extreme intensity that cannot be sustained for very long. Achieving this level is pointless because it can exhaust you and has no additional aerobic advantages.

Heart rate monitoring is, of course, the most common method of determining intensity.

The exercises given in this book can be done as a combination in your weight training routine or on alternate days. The decision is yours. You won't need to work out for hours to see results because these workouts are incredibly time-effective.

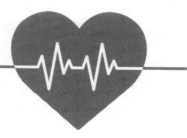

Chapter 3 : Aerobics: The Ultimate Fat Burning Workout

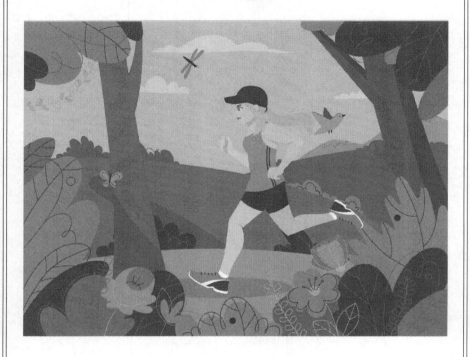

"Are you prepared to sweat and experience the burn? Prepare to explore the world of aerobics and reach a whole new fitness level!"

As we explore the thrilling and energizing world of aerobics, get your heart racing and your endorphins flowing. Aerobics offers several options to help you reach your fitness goals, from high-energy dance routines to low-impact workouts.

Learn about the science underlying aerobic exercise's capacity to enhance cardiovascular health, boost endurance, and promote general well-being. This chapter on aerobics is the ideal tool to help you get inspired and remain on track towards your goals, regardless of whether you are an experienced fitness enthusiast or are just beginning your journey towards well-being.

3.1 Welcome to Aerobics

I welcome you to the aerobics world, where ladies of all ages, physiques, and sizes assemble to move, groove, and work out! The various advantages of aerobic exercise for women—from higher mood and lower stress levels to improved cardiovascular health and increased stamina—will be covered in this chapter.

Aerobics is an enjoyable and successful way to reach your fitness objectives, regardless of whether you are a seasoned fitness enthusiast or a beginner trying to get in shape. There is something for everyone in the aerobics world: dance-inspired exercises, low-impact workouts, and high-intensity cardio sessions.

Now be ready to enter the great world of aerobics for ladies by lacing up your shoes, turning up the music, and getting your heart rate up. This engaging and inspiring exercise will surely appeal to you, whether your goals are to lose weight, tone your muscles, or feel more alive and invigorated.

Aerobics Vs. Anaerobic Exercises

Although aerobic and anaerobic workouts may sound similar, they are very different. Let me try to creatively convey it to you:

Imagine aerobic exercise as a steady, rhythmic dance that keeps your body grooving and moving for a long time. It is comparable to a marathon runner who keeps up a constant pace for long distances while relying on oxygen to fuel their muscles.

On the other hand, Anaerobic activities are similar to a series of short, explosive sprints that tax your body to the maximum. It is comparable to a powerlifter who uses the energy reserves in their muscles without any oxygen for a brief period of time while lifting a large weight.

Anaerobic activities focus on developing strength and power in quick bursts, whereas aerobic exercises are all about endurance and calorie burning over time. Both of them have a place in a fitness regimen that is well-rounded, but they have different objectives and employ various energy systems to get them.

So, knowing the difference between aerobic and anaerobic exercises can help you customize your workouts to meet your unique fitness goals, whether you are trying to increase your stamina or enhance your strength.

Consult Your Physician

Before beginning any workout program, I suggest you consult your doctor, especially if it has been a while since you last exercised. If you are new to exercising, consider speaking with a licensed personal trainer. They can advise you on additional activities that might be effective for you and offer tips for avoiding injuries while exercising.

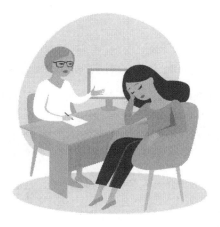

3.2 Aerobics Exercises

Some aerobics exercises include indoor exercises like an elliptical trainer, stair climbing, indoor rower, stationary bicycle, Stairmaster, treadmill, outdoor activities like cycling, cross-country skiing, inline skating, Nordic walking, jogging, football, soccer, and rugby, and indoor plus outdoor exercises like Kickboxing, jumping rope, swimming, circuit training.

Aerobics Strength Circuit

For this activity, you will need a firm chair and gym shoes. This exercise improves circulatory health, increases strength, and tones the main muscle groups. Pay close attention to your form during each exercise to ensure your safety. Maintain a reasonable heart rate throughout.

Time and frequency: 3-5 times a week for 15-25 minutes.

This exercise routine is meant to raise your heart rate. For one minute, do the following strengthening exercises:

Next, during your active rest, jog for 1 minute. Circuit one is complete. Between circuits, you get up to 5 minutes of rest. After that, relax your muscles.

Aerobics circuit training includes the following exercises:

Squats

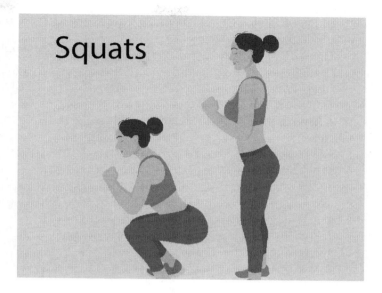

To begin:

◊ Stand with your feet apart and your toes pointing forward.

◊ Bend both legs and sit back until your bottom is at knee level.

◊ Your knees should go over the tips of your toes.

◊ Squeeze through your hips as you stand up.

◊ Do two to four sets of 25 reps each. If you can do more at the end of each set, you should do more reps.

- ◊ Keep proper form by maintaining shoulders back, chest high, and head up. Keep your torso from becoming horizontal to the earth.

- ◊ By expanding your pointing toes outward, you can try a variant of this standard squat. Your inner thighs will be the target of this technique.

Walking lunges

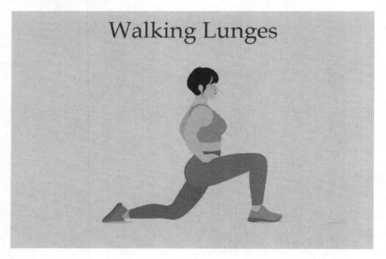

To begin:

- ◊ Put your feet apart and stand straight up.

- ◊ Step forward with the right leg, then bring your torso down until your back knee is either on the ground or almost on the ground.

- ◊ Using your front foot as a lever, raise yourself back up.

◊ Do the same with the left leg.

◊ Perform lunge for 30 seconds 2-4 times.

Maintain your trunk upright while doing this. Your lead knee should follow the shoelaces as you lower your torso and shoulders behind your toes.

Pushups

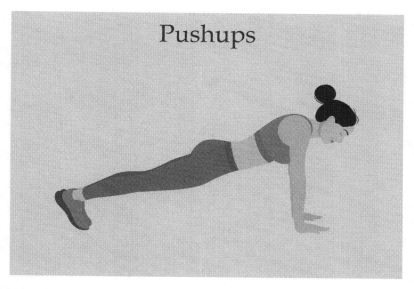

Pushups

To begin:

◊ Start with a position with your hands immediately beneath your shoulders, just outside shoulder width. Using your hands and toes, raise your body into the air. Avoid letting your hips drop, and keep your spine in neutral alignment.

◊ Return to a plank position right away by pressing your palms down.

◊ 5 sets of 15 reps should be done (adjust as needed).

Tip: Start with weight on the knees rather than the toes if this exercise is too difficult for you.

Crunches

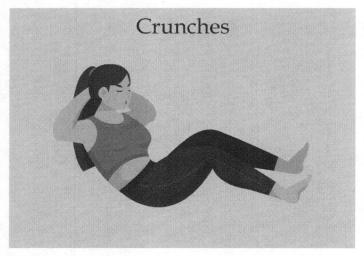
Crunches

To begin:

◊ A good place to start is on your back with your legs bent and your feet on the floor.

◊ Put both hands behind the head and put your arms out to the sides.

◊ Raise your shoulders and back by tightening your abs and bending your body up.

◊ Curl your elbows around your head.

◊ Don't lift yourself up with your muscles. Instead, fight the urge to use momentum.

◊ Maintain a distance between your chin and chest, the size of a golf ball.

◊ Slowly lower your body to activate as many muscles as possible.

◊ Complete five 25-rep sets.

◊ Don't use hands to tug on the head or neck. Your abs should be doing the work.

Jump Rope

You need a jump rope and gym footwear. Jumping rope improves agility, hand-foot coordination, and body alertness. Make sure your jump rope is sized appropriately for your height. Stand up and pull out the rope's handles. If the rope is too long, cut it or tie it so you don't trip over it.

Time and frequency: 3 to 5 times a week for 15 to 25 minutes.

Following a jump rope circuit is an excellent indoor or outdoor sport, but you will need lots of room. You should finish your circuit workout in 15 to 25 minutes.

◊   Rope. For 15 seconds, repeat this motion.

◊   Then, jog backwards for 15 seconds, and repeat this motion.

◊   Complete your set.

If you are a proficient exerciser, do this exercise for 30 seconds each while pausing for the same time between sets. It is recommended you complete the advanced circuit for 1 minute at a time, then take 60 seconds off.

3.3 A Perfect Aerobics Workout Plan

Here is a perfect aerobics plan for you:

Warm-Up:

To raise your heart rate and warm up your muscles, walk or lightly jog for 5–10 minutes.

Major Exercise:

3 sets of 12 repetitions on the squat. Starting with your feet shoulder-width apart, slowly squat down with straight back and knees.

Each set has ten pushes. Start in a plank position with your hands a little farther apart than shoulder-width apart. As you move your body toward the floor, keep your arms close to your body.

3 sets of 15 reps for crunches. Your hands should be behind your head while you lay on your back with your knees bent. Using your abdominal muscles, raise your shoulders off the ground as you slowly return to the beginning position.

3 sets of 10 walking lunge repetitions on each leg. Starting with your feet shoulder-width apart, step forward with one leg as far as possible, then lower your body into a lunge position. To stand back up, drive through your front heel. Next, repeat with the other leg.

Cooling Down

5 to 10 minutes of steady walking or stretching will help you gradually return to normal breathing and heart rate.

Always pay attention to your body and adjust the exercise to fit your fitness level and any potential physical restrictions. Regular use of this aerobic action plan can improve your strength, endurance, and general fitness.

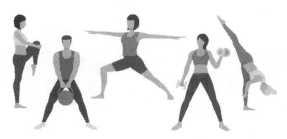

Chapter 4: Zumba: The Fun Way to Get Fit and Lean

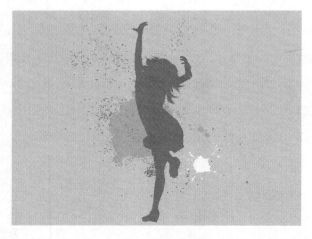

Are you ready for a celebration happening on international beats of the music? Soon, the space assumes the atmosphere of the dance. When I added Zumba to my workout routine, I noticed smiles, heard laughter, and experienced happiness. I felt wonderful when I realized that I was content and enjoying myself while exercising.

People are drawn to Zumba because they feel so happy when music is around, even those who do not enjoy working out. Yes, the main focus of Zumba classes is joy and fun. It's okay to memorize the steps. Enjoy yourself and see the outcomes.

4.1 Welcome to Zumba Party

Zumba is the most popular Latin dance fitness type worldwide. It combines dance steps to create an incredible workout. All of this takes place in a healthy, enjoyable, and party-like environment. Zumba "breaks all the exercise rules," as I like to say. It is formed when used as a dance-based workout. The routines have a well-defined structure, but you must follow them.

Move your body in time with the beat. In contrast to traditional aerobics, where you frequently move stiffly, jumping up legs straight out, Zumba routines involve using your entire body while moving to the music. You can trim your entire body shape with the help of this Zumba feature. It liberates your emotions and transforms exercise into a carefree activity. It gives you diversity and elevates your mood.

Many women claim they enjoy Zumba because it distracts them from their exercise routine. They enjoy Zumba because there is no pounding or jumping, making it gentler and safer on the joints. Women choose Zumba sessions because they are sick of gyms with intimidating equipment. They adore Zumba because it allows them to lose weight and inches without the normal setbacks associated with dieting or exercise boredom.

Humans have danced since the beginning to express their emotions, share their cultures, and free their souls. Both ancient Greek soldiers and cavemen engaged in it as battle preparation. The cavemen did it before the hunt to draw spiritual force from the prey. There are dances for weddings, welcomes, fertility, rain, and spiritual purposes. I can't think of a more commonplace way to celebrate life or respect our physical existence than via dance.

Dance belongs to health clubs just as much as in nightclubs or on stages. Anyone can participate in Zumba. I'm not a fan of this. Let free and enjoy yourself. The best part is that you lose weight and inches quickly. If you try, you can conquer your fear of dance, even if you find it daunting. It's just important to stay active and enjoy yourself.

The Bright Side of Zumba

Dancing is a fantastic form of exercise that is beneficial to uplifting your mood. But what exactly do Zumba and other forms of dancing accomplish for your body? What does it do to your mind, furthermore?

You will experience more body confidence, flexibility, and relaxation with Zumba, as well as the health advantages many exercise classes claim to provide but do not. Here is a closer examination of its advantages.

A Healthy Heart

Zumba is an aerobic activity since it uses a lot of huge muscle groups and is extended and rhythmic. Exercise that is "aerobic" improves the function of your cardio system. Literally, "aerobic" means "with oxygen." Your muscles need extra oxygen to function effectively when you exercise. Your respiration and heart rate increase due to trying to meet those demands. Carbon dioxide is exchanged for oxygen before being inhaled.

Sweating causes your body to release calories and fat. Zumba, or any dance, can increase your heart rate to anywhere between 120 and 160, strengthening and enduring your heart.

Moreover, aerobic exercise such as Zumba increases circulation, helps eliminate bad cholesterol buildup, strengthens your heart muscle, increases resting blood, and switches your body into fat-burning mode. It boosts metabolism and assists in blood pressure normalization.

Strength Training

Strength training is incorporated into Zumba routines. Resistance is used during strength training to improve a person's capacity to apply or withstand force. Strength training aims to condition, grow, preserve, and strengthen your muscles.

Muscles are your body's power plants. They support the body's conversion of food into fuel or metabolism. Your metabolism will function more quickly and, eventually, burn more calories. Strength training makes your engines bigger and better, which helps you lose fat more quickly and keep it off.

You stay young and active. Less muscle tissue means that calories that were once utilized to keep are now being stored as fat. This is avoided with strength training. Zumba helps you build muscles all around. Zumba stimulates various other muscles because it involves bending and moving in all directions.

We perform many crossover steps, which puts a lot of strain on the lower body, particularly the inner thighs. Your muscles will get stronger and more sculpted when you include some unique moves in your cardio workout.

Your joints may become stressed due to your movements during physical activity, sports, and even daily activities. Yet, strong muscles reduce this stress by helping to absorb shock and guard against impact damage. Further advantages of muscle conditioning include bettering posture, raising bone density, and lowering body fat.

There, you will discover some fun exercises that will help you strengthen, tone, and shape your muscles without using bulky weights or sophisticated equipment. Muscle-conditioning activities are enjoyable because we listen to great music as we exercise. Compared to performing a series of routine squats in a noisy, distracting gym, the music inspires you to work out harder and more intensely.

Attitude is more than a conceptual idea. Add spice and attitude to your motions by accentuating them with your hands, giving them a unique kick, or doing a sultry shimmy. Remember that Zumba's whole point is to let free and have fun.

Core Stability

Most people desire a firm, toned core to flaunt in bathing suits and bikinis, especially during the summer. But I can assure you that you will need more than hundreds of crunches for a short time. A mix of strength exercises, torso-toning aerobics, and a fun element are all essential components of an effective core workout. Zumba provides all three components. It exercises every muscle in your body. It excels at strengthening the core.

It takes core strength to build a gorgeous, toned figure from head to toe.

Consider this: Your core is where all motion originates. The remainder of your body will only be strong if your core is strong. Zumba naturally strengthens the stabilizing muscular body and lets you stand tall, as well as the muscles that assist in maintaining your belly get flat and strong.

Exercise with a higher heart rate, such as Zumba, is known to burn belly fat effectively. Compared to women of the same age and weight who have fat distributed in the lower body, those with abdominal fat are more likely to have higher triglyceride levels and a higher risk of dying from cardiovascular disease at a younger age. Hence, by reducing your waist, you get beautiful curves and improved health.

4.2 The Zumba's Moves: Getting Started

You will discover that Zumba is unlike any other workout program available. Remember that you can burn fat and tone your entire body with its constant, simple choreography without feeling like exercising!

If exercising is enjoyable and simple, you will continue doing it. The secret to managing your weight and maintaining good health over the long run is to stick with it and prioritize it in your life. Zumba routines combine aerobics with various motions that tone and sculpt the body. They are dynamic, exhilarating, and full of Latin and exotic music essences.

Zumba targets the heart, the most significant muscle, and the glutes, legs, arms, and abdominal. I think this combination of dance and shaping exercises will be an addicting and energizing workout.

Zumba workouts are a terrific decision you have made. As long as you use your muscles, your will gradually improve. Thus, it is crucial to keep your body moving. You may stay young and active by doing this.

Starting only requires a small bit of information and lots of enthusiasm. Here's how to get off to a good start.

Pick Up a New Lifestyle's Rhythm

If you are a beginner or haven't yet done much exercise in the past, start out slowly and don't push yourself over your ability or fitness level. Twice a week is an excellent place to start for someone with no prior experience in fitness.

Try to increase the length of each session over the coming weeks to at least three times for 45-60 minutes. Pay attention to your body's cues and see if you feel energized and like doing it!

You can undoubtedly accomplish more if you are physically fitter. Work at a rate just over your comfort zone while enabling you to carry on a conversation. Like any activity, stretch your muscles before and after to avoid cramping and damage.

Several women who try Zumba become so addicted that they attend classes or exercise at home each week for an hour. It's difficult to resist wanting to practice Zumba constantly because it's so much fun! But in all seriousness, your body does require recovery time. That may include doing out every day for some people or working out multiple days before taking a day or two off for others. Choose a routine that works with your lifestyle and body. Before starting any workout regimen, visit your doctor for a checkup. Moreover, dance, especially Zumba, is an aerobic activity.

Energize

Zumba exercises require a lot of energy. Therefore, you need to fuel yourself properly. Aside from that, feeling energized and well-fed can help you appreciate working out more. I have met a lot of exercisers who deliberately fast for three to four hours before their workouts. They forfeit the advantages of properly fed performance by doing this. When you run on fuel instead of fumes, your stamina and endurance will be much greater.

An essential refueling tactic is to have a healthy diet. It raises blood sugar and energy levels, enabling you to workout longer and harder. As a result, you will consume less energy. Breakfast also suppresses your appetite, so you will be less likely to treat yourself to high-calorie foods after working exercise. Chapter 7 provides some fantastic diet tips.

Another tactic is to eat a small snack an hour before you want to do Zumba to help you feel more energized than if you hadn't. This fueling regimen will greatly enhance your exercise performance. Avoid fatty foods like bacon, chips, fast food breakfasts, and other snacks and meals. Meals high in fat will make you sluggish.

Find Your Breath

Living is breathing! Our muscles, brain, and bones require oxygen to function. The body is effectively nourished by breathing in (also known as inspiration) and out (also known as expiration), improving movement, stamina, mental agility, and muscle coordination. While I was a professional dancer, I discovered that effective breath management might make the performance elegant. Keep your breathing deep and focus on the working muscles. You won't get tired since you will be consuming more oxygen.

Zumba Should be Complemented by other Forms of Exercise

The theme of the Zumba fitness program is freedom. Hence, you are to engage in activities other than Zumba. I enjoy lifting weights and running on the beach, for instance.

Yoga, Pilates, and various other workouts are becoming more popular than they were in the past.

I'm good with it if you want to include your exercise regimen. To enhance your Zumba experience, be open to new fitness opportunities and prepared to take advantage of them.

Entertain Yourself

I advise my pupils to move. You shouldn't exercise too vigorously or too lightly. The conversation test and heart rate monitoring are a few ways to determine how hard you are working out.

The "conversation test" is the easiest. It implies that you work out to talk to others. You should slow down if you need help to finish statements during exercise.

Nowadays, the simplest method to monitor your heartbeat during Zumba is by wearing a heart rate monitor. If you don't have one, you can take your pulse to check your heart rate the old-fashioned way. Find your pulse right away after working out at the radial artery. Start counting at 1 and continue for 10 seconds. Once you have your one minute, multiply it by 6 again.

Regarding heart rate, the accepted wisdom is to calculate your maximal heart rate (MHR). Just subtract your age from 220 to get there. As a result, your MHR is projected to be 190.

Make a Note

As you begin regularly practicing Zumba, you can anticipate seeing positive changes in your physique. The records should include startup details like height and weight measurements.

Before starting a fitness program, always have a certain weight goal in mind. In other words, aim for the weight you believe will make you look your best. Remember that there isn't such a thing as the "ideal" weight.

Zumba is a fitness program that draws participants in with a lively blend of dance techniques from genres like Salsa, Reggaeton, Cumbia, and Merengue. Let's discuss them one by one.

The Basic Salsa

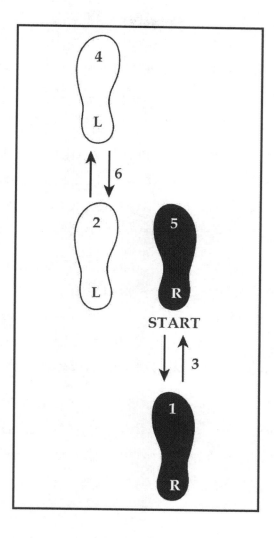

Salsa dancing is zesty, vibrant, and passionate, just like the term "salsa," which means "sauce," usually something hot and spicy. Salsa contains a rhythm of six steps spread over eight beats of music, and many of their movements are similar.

Salsa is fantastic because it is easy to learn. Because of its recent enormous growth in popularity, it is now danced in nightclubs. Salsa is a mix of Cuban, Puerto Rican, and African rhythms that combines a variety of Latin and Afro-Caribbean dances.

One of the key reasons salsa is most well-liked is that it's simple to learn. Although it might appear challenging at first, learning the fundamentals of salsa requires, at most, 10 to 15 minutes of practice.

One step comprises four beats, with one skipped between each step. Steps can be taken in circles, backwards and forwards, or from side to side. Maintaining a straight posture when dancing requires moving your hips as much as possible.

The dance can be performed either closed or open. Keep in mind that salsa has very few steps. The steps get smaller as the music gets faster, which is usually fairly rapid.

Directions:

Salsa has a wide variety of styles because it encourages creative improvisation. Nonetheless, the fundamental procedures are the same regardless of other styles. You should always start as a beginner.

Simple salsa moves for women are:

◊ Step backwards with your right foot. (beat one)

◊ As the foot is placed, the weight shifts to the left foot. (second beat)

◊ Put your right foot forward. (Pause for the final beat)

◊ Bring your left foot forward. (Again, on the first beat)

◊ Put your weight on your right foot. (two beats)

◊ Go backward with the left foot. (final third beat)

The Basic Cumbia

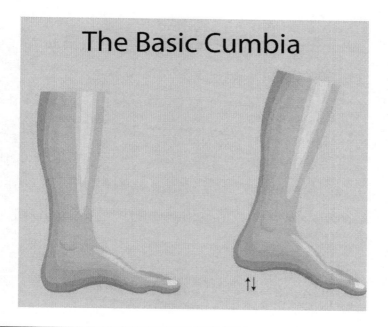

The Basic Cumbia

Cumbia is a lively and upbeat dance style incorporating movements such as shuffling and spinning. Cumbia is a favorite among dancers worldwide with its infectious rhythm and playful steps.

Start by slanting your body in the direction illustrated.

◊ Stand with feet together. Put equal amounts of weight on both feet.

◊ Start by moving the right leg. Keeping the left foot still, extend the right leg forward. Put your right foot forward and tap. Allow the right arm to swing backward while you swing your left arm forward.

◊ Afterward, tap the right foot and use your left leg throughout the procedure.

◊ Move your hips with your leg. Repeat this backward–forward pattern. Make a concerted effort to engage hips and core. The oblique muscles at the sides of the waist are effectively worked when you move with a modest waist twist.

◊ Repeat the sequence with the left leg and hands in the opposite direction.

I add fitness and directional modifications instead of arm variations when performing the Cumbia.

Cumbia Variation

Slightly lean forward. Try to extend the distance your leg travels back as far as possible. This exercise works your quads and abs.

The Reggaeton Basic

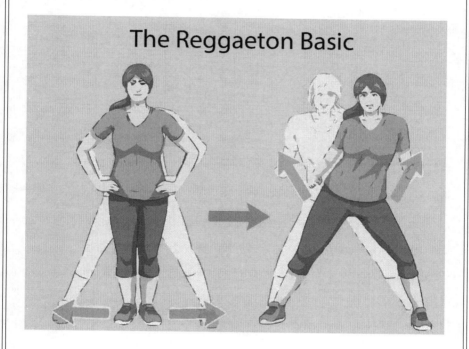
The Reggaeton Basic

The Reggaeton Basic is a popular modern dance style combining urban and traditional Latin dance elements. With its sexy and rhythmic movements, The Reggaeton Basic is a great way to get a full-body workout while having fun on the dance floor.

Directions:

◊ Place hands at sides and stand with feet together. This is a straightforward step-touch motion.

◊ Step with the right foot out to the right side.

◊ Then touch it with the left foot.

◊ With your left foot, take a step toward the left.

◊ Then touch it with the right foot.

◊ Move arms in the reverse directions from your body to add some reggaeton flair. You can perform a single step-touch followed by a double step-touch for a different pattern.

The Reggaeton Basic Variation

Make a right turn, perform a double step-touch, and then a single step-touch. Repeat while facing the other way. Repeat while pivoting to the side. To all four walls, repeat the maneuver while facing the front.

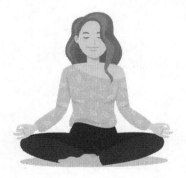

The Merengue March

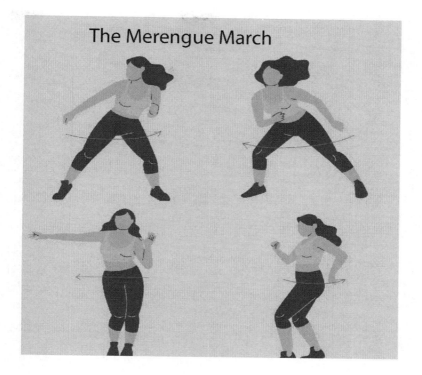

The Merengue March

The Merengue March is a fast-paced, lively dance style with quick, march-like steps. With its upbeat rhythm and playful movements, The Merengue March is a fun and energetic dance that is sure to get your heart pumping.

Direction:

◊ Place feet together and place arms at your sides to begin the march.

◊ Marching left and right should now begin.

◇ Let your hips swing in time with your foot motions naturally.

◇ Let knees slightly indent to engage hips.

◇ It's acceptable if your hips can't move very well; just keep marching.

◇ Your arms should move easily. Your left arm should go up when your right knee goes down, and your right arm should go up when your left knee goes down.

For the first arm version, put your arms outward toward the sides at about shoulder height.

◇ Straighten the right arm out after bending the right elbow and bringing the right hand to the chest.

◇ Straighten left arm out after bending the left elbow and bringing left hand to the chest. When you march, alternate this bending and straightening of arms. This arm movement has a waving appearance.

◇ Put arms up towards the ceiling in the second arm variation.

◇ Bring them back down to chest height after that.

◊ Bring arms to the front of the chest after that.

◊ Then, put arms by sides. Follow this pattern while marching to the music.

Directional Variation:

◊ Move march four steps forward and four steps backward. 4 steps ahead, 4 steps back, march to your right, then come back to the center.

◊ March to the rear, take 4 steps forward, 4 steps back, and then return to the middle.

◊ March four steps to the left, then four steps back, before returning to the middle.

Exercise Variation:

◊ When you march, spread your legs just over shoulder width apart while rocking your hips.

◊ Try one of the arm variants, or let your arms flow naturally.

◊ This action activates your core. Your quads should also experience it.

Chapter 5: Planks: The Secret to Strong and Toned Abs

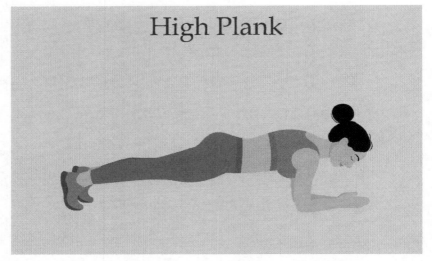
High Plank

Welcome to the world of planks- a straightforward but effective workout that may give you rock-solid strong and toned abs. We'll discuss the many advantages of planking in this chapter, including how it can help balance and posture and lower your risk of injury and back pain.

Planking is a bodyweight workout that requires no special equipment and can be performed anywhere, anytime. It entails maintaining a still position while keeping your spine straight and your body weight supported by your core muscles.

Planks have other advantages beyond only helping you develop a six-pack, such as raising your general fitness, improving your athletic performance, and even improving your mental health and general well-being.

This chapter is the definitive guide to mastering the art of planking, whether you are a novice trying to incorporate planks into your training regimen or a seasoned fitness enthusiast looking to push your core strength to the next level as you learn how planks can help you get strong, toned abs. Prepare to feel the heat!

5.1 Welcome to a Killer Core

Plank is a quick and simple exercise that may give women a killer core. It is a common option for ladies who want to exercise at home or on the go because it is a bodyweight exercise that needs no equipment and can be performed anywhere.

With the arms straight and the body in the straight line, the plank is a static exercise that requires holding the body in a position like the top of a push-up. The abdominals, obliques, and lower back are the core muscles typically worked during this exercise.

Planks provide numerous advantages for women. The core muscles can be strengthened and toned, which can aid with posture, lower back problems, and general fitness. A strong core can also make it easier and less dangerous for women to conduct daily tasks like lifting heavy things or transporting groceries.

Planks can help increase whole-body strength and stability and strengthen the core. Several distinct muscular groups, including the arms, shoulders, and legs, are used during this exercise, which can increase general fitness and lower the chance of injury.

Planks have the advantage of being easily adapted to match women's various fitness levels and objectives. Beginners might hold a simple plank position for 30 to 1 minute. At the same time, more experienced ladies might add variants like side planks or plank jacks to enhance the difficulty level and focus on other areas of the core.

Planks can also help women become more physically active and healthy overall. This activity is an excellent addition to any fitness regimen because it can improve endurance, speed up metabolism, and lower stress levels.

5.2 Fun Plank Variations

Planks are incredibly resilient and useful for women. Planks are a multipurpose exercise that trains more than 20 muscles, including the shoulders, arms, back, legs, and glutes and your core. Even better, planks allow you to strengthen your core dangers of back pain and overworked hip flexors associated with conventional sit-ups. Start with the simple workouts to learn how to perform the fundamental plank correctly, then go to interesting variations.

Forearm Plank

- Start with the tabletop position and your feet hip-width apart. (see the image at the start of chapter.)

- Elbows should be straight to the shoulders as you lower each forearm to the ground one at a time. Make hard fists or firmly place your palms on the ground.

- Raise both knees and straighten your legs into a position while contracting your glutes and stabilizing your core.

- Maintain for 45 seconds. 3 sets are recommended.

High Plank

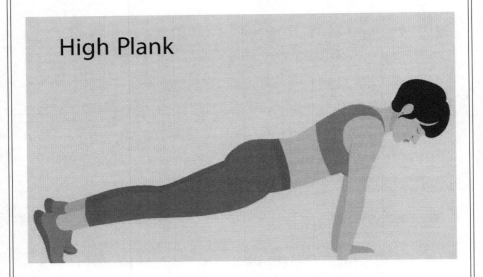

High Plank

Start with the tabletop position with your feet hip-width apart, your knees bent under your hips and your hands directly beneath your shoulders. Keep your elbows straight, your shoulders, and lower one forearm at a time to the ground. Put your palms on the ground or make soft fists.

Squeeze your glutes together and engage your core as you lift knees off the ground and straighten your legs. Actively push off the ground, keeping your body straight from head to heels.

Take a 45-second hold. Make 3 sets.

Knee Plank

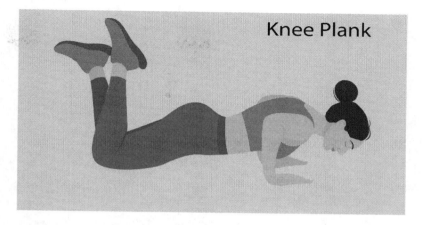

Knee Plank

Lay on your right side with both legs to the left side and your feet stacked. Your right elbow should be on the floor next to your right shoulder.

Activate your core, lift your hips and knees off the ground with your right foot and elbow and raise your left arm towards the ceiling simultaneously.

Take a 45-second hold. Alternate sides; repeat. Make 3 sets.

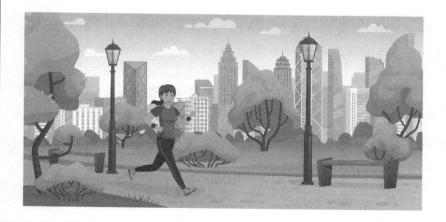

Side Plank

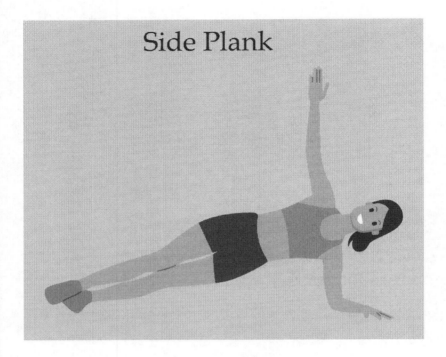

Side Plank

Starting from a tabletop position on the floor, place your hands beneath your shoulders; knees bent and under your hips. Lower one forearm toward the ground while keeping your elbows close to your shoulders. Make gentle fists or place your palms on the floor.

As you straighten your legs into a plank position, tighten your glutes and tense your abs. Maintain a head-to-toe alignment with your body.

Hold for 45 seconds. Create three sets.

Reverse Plank

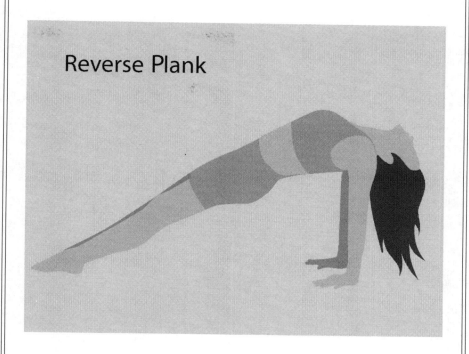

Reverse Plank

Put your palms—with fingers spread widely—slightly outside and behind your hips on the ground.

Lift your upper body and hips up and press down on your hands. Look up at the sky as you do this. Straighten your arms and legs. From your head to your feet, your whole body is in a straight line. Hold this position for 30 seconds.

Bring your spine and hips back down to the ground to get back to where you started.

Mountain Climber Plank

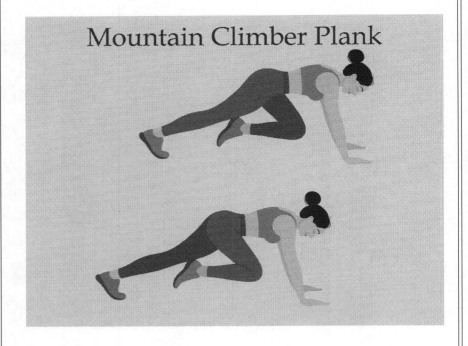

When you first begin, attempt the traditional exercise variation:

Lie on your back in a plank position with your weight equally distributed between your toes and hands.

Your head should be straight, back in flat position, and your hands should be about shoulder-width apart.

Pull the right knee as far into your chest as you can.

Keep your hips down and use your knees to sprint as swiftly and far as you can. Alternately inhale and exhale with each leg movement.

While moving, control your breathing. Don't forget to breathe.

Plank Shoulder Taps

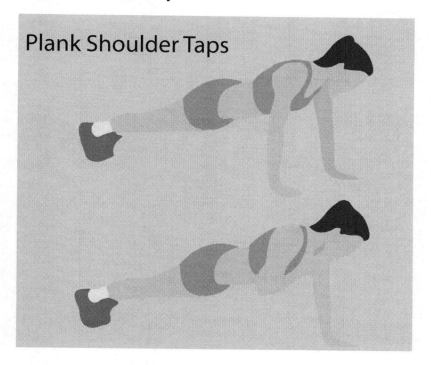

Start with the tabletop position with your feet hip-width apart, your knees under your hips, and your hands directly beneath your shoulders.

Raise your knees off the ground and get on your palms while contracting your core and squeezing your glutes together.

Actively push off the ground, keeping your body straight from your head to your heels. This is where everything begins.

While maintaining a square posture, lift your hand and touch your left shoulder. Lifting the left hand, tap the right shoulder with the lower right hand. Repeat.

Alternate continuously for 45 seconds. Make 3 sets.

Up Down Plank

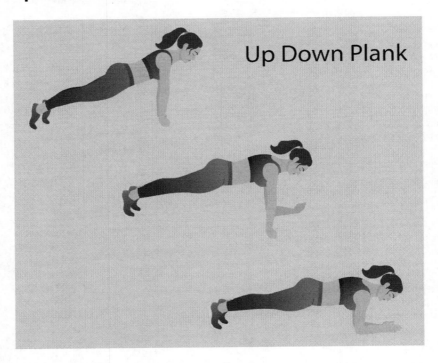

Up Down Plank

Start with the tabletop position with your feet hip-width apart, your knees bent under your hips and your hands directly beneath your shoulders.

Raise both knees and get to plank position on your palms while contracting your core and squeezing your glutes together.

Actively push off the ground, keeping your body straight from head to heels. This is where everything begins.

While keeping your hips aligned, bring your left elbow into the plank before lowering your right elbow. Put your right hand on your right shoulder and your left hand on your left shoulder.

Now, lower your left elbow toward the floor and then your right elbow to make a forearm plank. Put your left hand on your left shoulder and your right hand on your right shoulder.

Then alternate for a further 60 seconds. Make 3 sets.

Take a plank challenge and do one plank position daily. Remember to listen to your body and take breaks as needed. Good luck with the challenge!

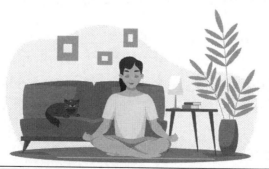

Chapter 6: Maximizing Your Results with Strength Training

Strength training is an exercise that uses resistance to cause muscular contraction. Anybody wishing to shed weight or enhance their athletic ability should consider this sort of exercise. But it's critical to have a firm grasp of the underlying concepts and methods to get the most out of strength training.

The advice in this chapter will help you reach your fitness objectives, regardless of whether you are a beginner just getting started with strength training or an experienced athlete trying to improve your performance. So let's explore the realm of strength training right now!

6.1 Arms

The muscles in the front and rear of your arm are divided into two categories. The biceps brachii, often known as the bis, is the most prominent muscle on the front of the arm. Though less well-known than the biceps, the brachialis is no less significant. Flexing the elbow is the major purpose of it.

The triceps brachii, often known as the tris, is the main muscle on the back of the arm. The tris is a tendon that connects to the ulna, a bone in the forearm, and has three unique heads: a long and a lateral head. The triceps' three heads straighten the elbow from a bent posture.

Tight, toned arms are a sign of success for sports enthusiasts and fitness freaks alike. Sculpting all the proper regions necessitates focused efforts because daily tasks do present some resistance. These exercises maintain long, slim, and strong biceps and triceps arms.

Side-Lying Push-Up

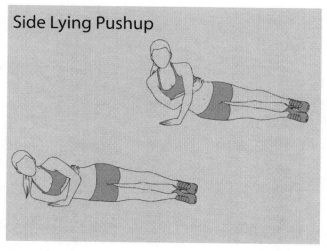

Side Lying Pushup

Follow the instructions:

◊ Lay on your side and cross one arm over your abdominals.

- ◊ Your elbow creates a straight angle in this position.
- ◊ Place your other hand on the ground directly in front of you.
- ◊ Lift your other arm entirely off the ground by pressing through your arm until it is almost straight.
- ◊ Return to the starting position slowly.
- ◊ Continue until you succeed, then switch sides.
- ◊ Use the exercises listed here to perform triceps workouts twice each week. Change the movements and the sequence each time to confuse and stimulate the muscle.

Bench Dip

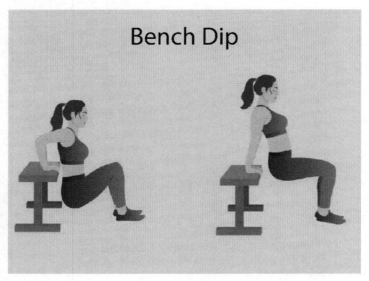

Follow the instructions:

◊ Place your feet firmly on the ground and sit upright on the longest side of the bench.

◊ Palms facing down, grab the seat immediately in front of your hips.

◊ Lift your glutes away from the bench, then slowly and deliberately drop yourself until your elbows are at a 90-degree angle.

◊ Set your feet on a second bench to make the challenge harder.

6.2 Chest

A physique that turns heads requires more than just toned thighs and abs. The chest is among the largest body components. It is essential for muscle balance and upper-body strength. Utilize it to the maximum in your effort to shape your torso.

The pectoralis major, often known as the pectorals or pecs, is the main muscle of the chest. It is a substantial muscle with two heads: the sternocostal head is located on the lower and middle chest, while the clavicular head is located on the upper region of the chest.

Ball Push-Up

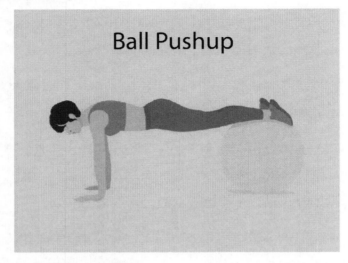

Follow the instructions:

◊ Put the ball beneath your shins and start doing push-ups with your hands slightly wider than shoulder-width apart.

◊ Maintain a flat back so that your entire body is in a straight position.

◊ Do not let your lower back arch.

◊ Instead, merely lower your chest as much as your comfort level allows.

◊ While you press back up, maintain your chest raised.

◊ If you are a novice, place the ball nearer to the hips for added support.

◊ As you get more accustomed to the exercise, gradually move the ball down your legs.

Ball Dumbbell Press

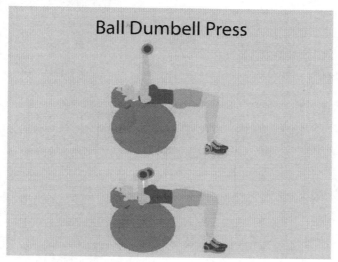

Follow the instruction:

◊ Lie while facing the ball with both knees slightly bent at 90 degrees angle to fully support your neck, upper body, and head.

◊ Keep your upper body and thighs parallel to the floor.

◊ Hold the dumbbell above the shoulders with the palms towards your feet, and squeeze your chest to raise your arms.

◊ Slowly bring your arms back to parallel positions.

6.3 Legs

Everyone aspires to have an attractive lower half with elegant curves. But more than just being aesthetically pleasing, our legs must also be capable of carrying us to our desired location. The key is muscle equilibrium from top to bottom.

Hip Raise

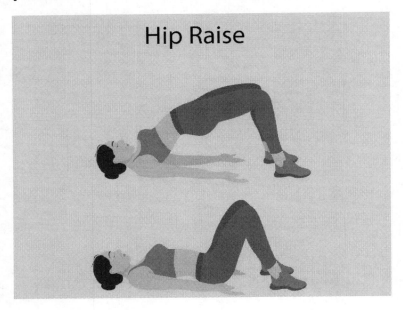

Follow the instruction:

◊ Put your feet on a slightly elevated surface while lying face up with knees bent.

◊ Place a dumbbell on your lower abs and slowly raise the hips toward the sky while pushing your knees away from your body.

◊ Your shoulder and feet will feel the weight of your body.

◊ Squeeze your glutes, hold them for a second.

◊ Gradually return to original position.

Calf Raise

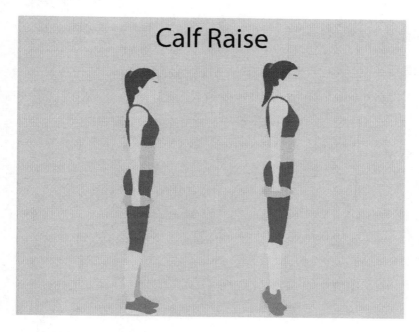

Follow the instruction:

◊ Grab a chair or a wall for support as you maintain a straight posture with both feet apart.

◊ Slowly elevate your heels to balance your weight on the feet.

6.4 Upper body

There are no shortcuts to anything worth going, as you have probably already heard. Hence, you must become stronger by working out more if you like to bulk up your back, chest, arms, and shoulders and improve the appearance of your entire body as a result.

Bent-Over Row

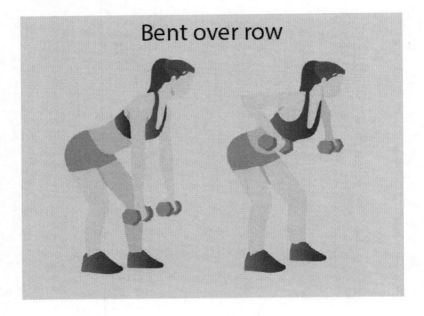

Follow the instruction:

◊ Standing with both feet apart and knees bent, hold the ball out in front of the body with both hands while keeping your arms straight.

◊ With your back flat and your head in a neutral position, tighten your abs and bend forward at the hips.

◊ Squeeze your shoulder together while bringing the ball in towards your abs.

◊ Hold for one minute, then go backward.

Ball Throw

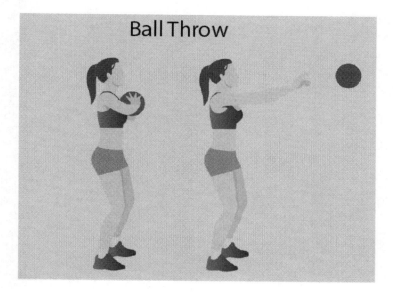

Follow the instruction:

◊ Hold the ball above your chest as you lay face up.

◊ Toss the ball directly above you into the air with extended arms; catch it as it descends and bring it back to your chest.

◊   As you advance, raise the throw's height.

6.5 Lower Body

You probably fantasize about having toned, tight thighs and defined glutes. Combine these exercises with upper-body training to forge a stunning physique.

Tuck Jump

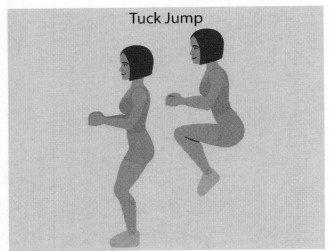

Tuck Jump

Follow the instruction:

◊   Jump as high as you can, starting from a "ready" position with your arms extended.

◊   Reduce the time your feet are on the ground by jumping directly into the next one when you touch down.

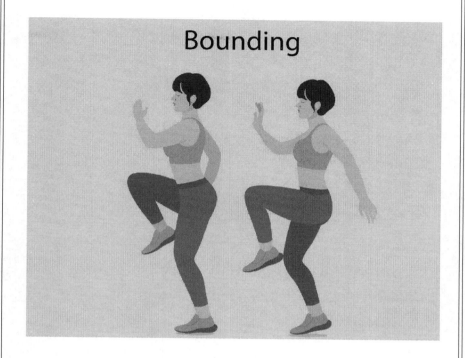

Bounding

Follow the instruction:

◊ Consider this exercise to be a vigorous kind of skipping.

◊ You skip, pushing your knees forward and lifting your body high and far forward.

6.6 Full-body Plan

You should execute a full-body plan thrice at home to maintain your body's fitness. You will work on all primary muscle groups every time you exercise. For each muscle group, perform a single exercise. Every time you exercise, you train your complete body; further exercises are unneeded and may even be harmful.

Extending your workout beyond the prescribed schedule will only hinder your body's ability to recover, which can eventually result in overtraining. Keep in mind that less is more when it comes to exercising.

Certain muscles serve as main movers, while others work as synergists or stabilizers. Even some muscles exist only to read and correct body posture changes to maintain balance. Exercises that involve several joints simulate daily activities that call for your muscles to work together as a linked chain.

Multi-joint activities have two advantages.

First, such activities offer a productive way to exercise. Moreover, it maximizes your metabolic rate. More muscle use results in more calorie burnout. The result is increased lean body mass and improved general fitness and health perception.

Not all muscle groups, however, are suitable for multi-joint activities.

This full body exercise plan targets specific muscles while also providing variation for the larger muscle groups. The interaction of this plan causes a variety of proprioceptive reactions that train your body to function effectively in a variety of diverse contexts. Since most real-world activities are performed on stable ground, stable-surface training is given more attention.

Sets

Each exercise should be done three times. Execute the sets using the classic block method. This means that after performing one set of an exercise, you will rest before performing your second and third sets. Go on to the next exercise after completing your third set, and complete the succeeding sets similarly.

You could be pondering the necessity of performing three sets of each workout.

Despite all, some fitness experts still support the idea that one set is all needed to fully engage you that further sets are unnecessary.

I'm sorry, but science disagrees. Studies have consistently proven that multiple-set protocols are preferable in developing muscle strength and development, even while single-set regimens undoubtedly make good use of time and can yield modest effects. The overwhelming research: You must train with many sets to maximize outcomes and prevent plateauing: a point where you fitness progress is halted.

You get into your subconscious by performing an exercise repeatedly, creating an important connection between the mind and the muscle. The early stages of training, before your body grows accustomed to creating synchronized motions between joints, are when this exercise is very crucial. Exercises only become second nature after consistent repetition and focusing on honing your ability and power.

We are all aware that life might occasionally interfere with exercise. You might occasionally run out of time and need help to complete a whole exercise. In these cases, reduce the total sets to ensure your body gets a workout. It's better to get little exercise than none at all.

Always aim to complete the entire amount of sets, and only make concessions when they are required.

Repetitions

For each set, there are 15-20 repetitions. Your body will be better able to handle any physical obstacle you may face, whether it lasts an hour or more.

This exercise plan carefully divides repetitions into days focusing on strength, power, and endurance. The first day aims for 15-20 repetitions, the second day has a moderate range of 8-12 reps, and the third has a low range of 4-6 reps. Use these ranges as broad recommendations rather than strict rules. You are allowed to occasionally deviate from the recommended range. Little changes won't hurt and may even benefit you by forcing your body to adapt to new challenges.

The repetition routine has one restriction: If you stick to greater reps until you feel comfortable. This is crucial when using free weights because they call for more technical execution. Get accustomed to how a movement feels. Put it into your unconscious mind. After developing muscle memory, you can start using different repetition ranges, moving to moderate-rep and low-rep sets.

Rest

Take a 30-90-second break between sets. Repetition and rest typically have an inverse connection. With greater reps, you need less rest, while lower reps need more rest.

Short rest intervals are advantageous because high-rep sets increase muscular endurance. This exercise strains the slow-twitch, fatigue-resistant muscle fibers needed for aerobic activity. Take a brief break of about 30 seconds between sets to collect your breath.

Your body will eventually become used to the quick speed, and you won't experience any problems switching from one set to the next.

On the other hand, higher rep sets need less recovery to fully refill your body's energy reserves. All your body's resources must be used to devote maximum lift since lower-rep sets to increase strength and power. Depending on several physical circumstances, you can need up to 2 minutes. In conclusion, wait to go on until you are certain that you are prepared for your best.

Intensity

Your goal should be to allow your body to adjust to the plan and the demands of weight training. It's comparable to how you'd swim in a chilly pool. Without first testing the water, would you cannonball from the diving board?

While it is understandable that you want to see results quickly, overworking can stress you a lot.

The final result is impaired outcomes or, worse yet, a training injury. As a result, pick a starting weight that is moderately difficult but only demands a little work to complete the set.

Use the progressive overload once your body has gotten used to the exercise. Make sure the weight you employ is suitably difficult. Push yourself to the point of momentary muscle failure during the final set or the point at which you are unable to perform another repeat. This will guarantee continual advancement and aid in avoiding stagnation.

6.6 7-Days Workout Plan

Here's a 7-days workout plan for women that incorporates aerobics, planks, Zumba, and strength training exercises:

Day 1: Aerobics, Planks, and Strength Training

- Warm-up: 10 minutes of cardio (walking or jogging)

- Aerobics: 20 minutes of moderate-intensity cardio (brisk walking, cycling, or elliptical)

- Planks: 30-second planks (3 sets), with a 30-second rest in between each set

- Strength Training: 12 reps of strength training exercises. (3 sets)

- Cool-down: Do stretching for 5 minutes

Day 2: Zumba and Strength Training

- Warm-up: 10 minutes of cardio (walking or jogging)

- Zumba: 30 minutes of Zumba dance workout

- Strength Training: 12 reps of strength training exercises. (3 sets)

- Cool-down: Do stretching for 5 minutes

Day 3: Planks, Aerobics, and Strength Training

- Warm-up: 10 minutes of cardio (walking or jogging)

- Planks: 45-second planks (3 sets), with a 30-second rest in between each set

- Aerobics: 20 minutes of moderate-intensity cardio (brisk walking, cycling, or elliptical)

- Strength Training: 12 reps of strength training exercises. (3 sets)

- Cool-down: Do stretching for 5 minutes

Day 4: Zumba and Strength Training

- Warm-up: 10 minutes of cardio (walking or jogging)

- Zumba: 30 minutes of Zumba dance workout

- Strength Training: 12 reps of strength training exercises. (3 sets)

- Cool-down: Do stretching for 5 minutes

- Day 5: Planks, Aerobics, and Strength Training

- Warm-up: 10 minutes of cardio (walking or jogging)

- Planks: 60-second planks (3 sets), with a 30-second rest in between each set

- Aerobics: 20 minutes of moderate-intensity cardio (brisk walking, cycling, or elliptical)

- Strength Training: 12 reps of strength training exercises. (3 sets)

- Cool-down: Do stretching for 5 minutes

Day 6: Zumba and Strength Training

- Warm-up: 5 minutes of light cardio (walking or jogging)

- Zumba: 30 minutes of Zumba dance workout

- Strength Training: 12 reps of strength training

exercises. (3 sets)

- Cool-down: Do stretching for 5 minutes

Day 7: Rest day

- Take a break and let your body recover from the previous workouts.

- Adjust the workout plan according to your fitness level and preferences. And most importantly, have fun while getting fit!

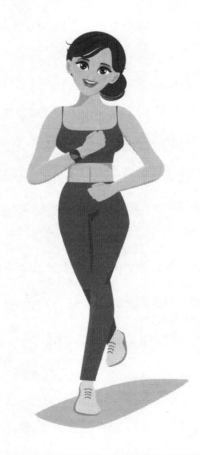

Chapter 7: Diet for a Lean Body

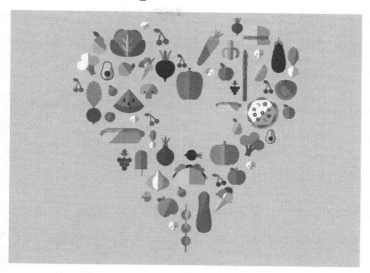

For a lean body and to lose weight, a healthy diet should include whole, nutrient-dense foods that give your body the vitamins, macronutrients. and minerals it needs. Here are some helpful tips that will assist you eat well to lose weight:

Eat a lot of fruit and veggies: These foods have a lot of fiber, which gives you important nutrients.

Choose protein sources with less fat: Chicken, fish, turkey, eggs, beans, tofu and peas are all good options.

Eat good fats: Nuts, seeds, bananas, and olive oil are all good sources of healthy fats.

Control portion sizes: Pay attention to how much you eat and listen to the body's signals when it tells you it's hungry or full.

Drink water: Drink a lot of water to keep your weight at a healthy level, which can help you feel less hungry.

Consider tracking your food intake: Keeping a food journal or using a tracking app can help you monitor food intake and ensure you eat a balanced diet.

Remember, a healthy diet is just part of a weight loss plan. Be sure to incorporate regular physical activity and prioritize sleep and stress management to support your overall health and weight loss goals.

7 Days Diet Plan for a Lean Body

Here is a sample 7-Day diet plan for a lean body and weight loss:

Day 1:

Breakfast: Omelet made with spinach, 2 eggs, and diced tomato, served with toast.

Snack: 1 medium apple with some almonds.

Lunch: Grilled chicken, mixed vegetables (broccoli, carrots, and peppers) and brown rice.

Snack: 2 small container of Greek yogurt with banana and honey.

Dinner: Salmon (baked) fillet with green beans and a side salad (lettuce, cucumber, cherry tomatoes, and balsamic vinegar dressing).

Day 2:

Breakfast: Greek yogurt and sliced peaches.

Snack: 1 small cottage cheese container with sliced cucumber and a handful of cherry tomatoes.

Lunch: Grilled shrimp with mixed vegetables (zucchini, squash, and onions) and quinoa.

Snack: 2 small handful of cashews and 1 small apple.

Dinner: Turkey meatballs with marinara sauce served over spaghetti squash with a side salad (lettuce, cucumber, cherry tomatoes, and vinaigrette dressing).

Day 3:

Breakfast: Overnight cereal made with rolled oats, chia seeds, unsweetened almond milk, and sliced strawberries.

Snack: 1 small container of hummus.

Lunch: Grilled chicken, roasted sweet potatoes and a side salad (lettuce, cucumber, cherry tomatoes, and lemon dressing).

Snack: 2 small container of plain Greek yogurt with diced mango and a sprinkle of cinnamon.

Dinner: Lean beef, carrots, snow peas, and broccoli stir-fried with brown rice.

Day 4:

Breakfast: Toast made with 1 slice of whole-grain bread, mashed avocado, and sliced tomato.

Snack: 1 small handful of walnuts and 1 small apple.

Lunch: Grilled chicken, quinoa, and Brussels sprouts that had been roasted.

Snack: Two small containers of cottage cheese with strawberry slices and honey drizzled on top.

Dinner: Baked cod fillet with roasted asparagus and a side salad (lettuce, cucumber, cherry tomatoes, and vinaigrette dressing).

Day 5:

Breakfast: Protein smoothie made with unsweetened almond milk, frozen mixed berries, and whey protein powder.

Snack: 1 small container of Greek yogurt with sliced peaches and a sprinkle of granola.

Lunch: Grilled chicken with sweet potatoes and mixed vegetables (carrots, bell peppers, and onions).

Snack: 2 small handful of almonds and 1 small pear.

Dinner: Baked chicken breast with roasted green beans and a side salad (lettuce, cucumber, cherry tomatoes, and balsamic vinegar dressing).

Day 6:

Breakfast: Scrambled eggs with spinach and sliced avocado.

Snack: 1 small container of hummus with sliced cucumber and a handful of cherry tomatoes.

Lunch: Grilled shrimp with roasted asparagus and brown rice.

Snack: 2 small container of plain Greek yogurt with diced pineapple and a sprinkle of cinnamon.

Dinner: Baked salmon fillet with roasted Brussels sprouts and a side salad (lettuce, cucumber, cherry tomatoes, and vinaigrette dressing).

Day 7:

Breakfast: 1 cup oatmeal, 3 egg whites, half cup strawberries

Snack: 1 ½ cup of green vegetables, 10 oz. of chicken breast

Lunch: Potato (baked), 1 ½ cup of green vegetables, and 8 oz. of turkey

Snack: 1 cup of berries

Dinner: 7 oz. Lean steak and 5-8 stalks of asparagus

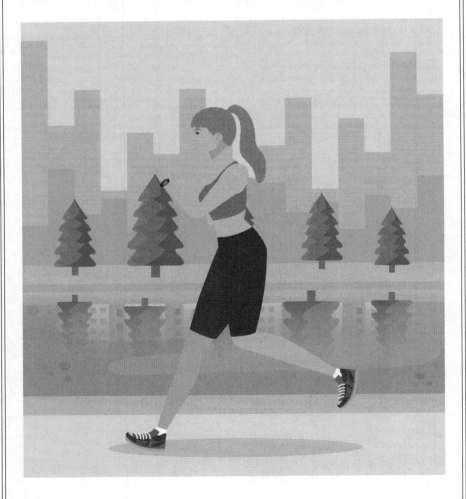

Conclusion

The world of fitness has seen a significant shift in recent years, with more and more women embracing various workout routines as part of their lifestyle. In this book on women's workout, we have explored some of the most popular and effective workouts for women, including Zumba, aerobics, planks, and strength training. While each workout has its unique benefits, they all share a common goal: to help women achieve a healthier and more active lifestyle.

Aerobics is a classic workout that has been popular for decades. This exercise involves rhythmic movements that increase the heart rate and improve cardiovascular health. Aerobics can also help to burn calories and reduce body fat, making it an effective workout for weight loss. With various types of aerobics, such as step aerobics, dance aerobics, and water aerobics, there is something for everyone.

Zumba has gained immense popularity recently, with women of all ages joining the dance party to shed those extra pounds and improve their overall health. This fun and high-energy workout combine various dance styles with music, making it easy for anyone to follow along. One of the unique aspects of Zumba is that it offers a full-body workout while allowing participants to let loose and have fun.

Planks are a form of isometric exercise that targets the body's core muscles. This workout involves holding the body in a straight line for as long as possible, engaging the core muscles and strengthening them. Planks are an excellent exercise for women who want to improve their posture, reduce lower back pain, and enhance their fitness.

While these workouts are all effective in their ways, it's essential to find a workout routine that works for you. Whether you prefer to dance your way to fitness with Zumba, engage in high-energy aerobics, strengthen your core with planks, or build muscle with strength training, the most important thing is to stay consistent and committed.

In conclusion, the world of women's fitness is diverse and exciting, offering a range of workouts to suit different preferences and goals. Incorporating workouts like Zumba, aerobics, planks, and strength training into your fitness routine can improve your health, boost your energy levels, and enhance your overall well-being.

Made in United States
Orlando, FL
15 November 2024

53930786R00061